Eating For Your Blood Type

Unlocking The Secret To A Healthier You

By

Marcus Frye

Table Of Contents

Introduction:

Have you ever questioned why some diets are immensely effective for some people while failing for others? It's possible that our blood type holds the key. The blood type diet hypothesis postulates that various blood types have been developed to suit various diets. Hence, eating in accordance with your blood type may help you achieve your healthiest and most satisfied state.

We shall look into the idea of adjusting your diet based on ouryour blood type in this book. We will examine the science of the blood type diet, including how it functions and the foods that are best for each blood type.

We will debunk common myths about the blood type diet and offer evidence-based explanations of how it can improve your health. Understanding your blood type and how it affects your food is a crucial step towards accomplishing your health objectives, whether you're trying to get in shape, increase your energy, or fend off chronic diseases.

Therefore, if you're prepared to learn which foods are ideal for your blood type, let's get started and discover

how tailoring your diet may be the
key to maximizing your health.

Chapter 1

Introduction To Blood Type Diet.

The idea that a single dietary strategy can be effective for everyone, despite their individual characteristics, is known as the "one size fits all" diet. Although many diets claim to work for everyone, this concept has gained a lot of traction in the field of nutrition.

The blood type diet theory is one such diet that allegedly caters to individual needs. According to this diet, a person's blood type should dictate what they consume in order to improve their health and wellness. An overview of the blood type diet idea, its background, and the debate around its efficacy will be given in this chapter.

According to the blood type diet theory, each blood type has unique nutritional needs since different blood types originated in various environments and at various times. This belief states that blood type O is the oldest blood type and that individuals with this blood type are referred to as "hunters" who require a high-protein diet rich in meat. Blood type A is supposed to have evolved later and is associated with "cultivators" who should eat a mostly vegetarian diet. People with blood type B are referred to as "nomads" and are advised to eat a varied diet that includes both animal- and plant-based foods. Blood type B is thought to have originated in nomadic tribes. Last but not least, blood type AB is assumed to have developed more recently and is a blend of blood types A and B, necessitating a diet that includes both.

According to the blood type diet idea, eating a diet specific to your blood type will improve your health, ward off disease, and help you keep a healthy weight. Based on your blood type, the diet suggests particular foods to eat and stay away from. It also offers recommendations for meal planning and serving sizes.

Dr. Peter D'Adamo, a naturopathic doctor, initially put forth the blood type diet notion in his 1996 book "Eat Well 4 Your Type." Our blood type is a predictor of our ancestry and the eating patterns of our ancestors, according to Dr. D'Adamo's theory. He asserted that we can improve our health and prevent disease by eating according to our blood type.

The blood type diet notion acquired a lot of traction since many people claimed that by following the diet, their health had significantly improved. Some nutrition experts have, however, criticized the hypothesis, claiming that there is no scientific data to back up the assertions made by the blood type diet theory.

While being generally accepted, the blood type diet theory has received harsh criticism from nutritionists for being unsupported by research. There is no evidence to back up the claims made by the blood type diet theory, according to a review of the scientific literature on the topic that was published in the American Journal of Clinical Nutrition in 2013.

The blood type diet theory has its detractors who claim that the suggestions provided by the diet are based on an incorrect knowledge of human physiology and evolution. They contend that there is no scientific evidence to support the idea that our blood type is a predictor of our nutritional needs and that adopting a diet specific to our blood type will improve our health.

One such diet is the blood type diet theory, which contends that a person's diet should be based on their blood type in order to promote their health and welfare.

Chapter 2

Blood Types: The Science Behind Them.

The presence or lack of certain antigens on the surface of red blood cells is used to identify blood types. Blood comes in four main categories: A, B, AB, and O. The unique antigens found on the surface of red blood cells help identify each blood type.

Red blood cells from people with blood type A contain the A antigen. Moreover, their plasma has antibodies to the B antigen. A1 and A2 are the two subtypes of blood type A, with A1 being the most prevalent. Heart disease and some cancers are known to be more common in those with blood type A.

Red blood cells from people with blood type B contain the B antigen. In their plasma, they have antibodies against the A antigen. Less people have blood type B than type A, and more people in Asia have blood type B than in Europe or the Americas. Pancreatic cancer is reported to be more common in people with blood type B.

Red blood cells of people with blood type AB contain both the A and B antigens. In their plasma, they don't have any antibodies to either A or B antigens. Just about 4% of people have blood type AB, making it the least common of the four blood types. Blood clots are thought to be more likely to form in those with blood type AB.

Red blood cells of people with blood type O do not contain the A or B antigens. Their plasma contains antibodies to both the A and B antigens. Around 45% of people have blood type O, making it the most prevalent blood type. It is well established that those with blood type O are less likely to experience heart disease and pancreatic cancer.

Given that some people think specific blood types are better suited to particular types of diets, blood type may be a factor in determining dietary requirements. According to the hypothesis underlying this notion, eating according to one's blood type might enhance general health and lower the risk of certain diseases because different blood types evolved in response to diverse dietary requirements.

For instance, it is believed that blood type A individuals benefit most from a vegetarian diet, whereas blood type O individuals are considered to benefit most from a high-protein, low-carbohydrate diet. Yet, there is little solid scientific evidence in favor of the claim that dietary requirements can be accurately predicted based on blood type. Although it is true that various environmental forces, such as diet, led to the evolution of distinct blood types, there is no conclusive proof that eating according to one's blood type is essential for good health.

The presence or lack of specific antigens on the surface of red blood cells determines blood type, and each blood type is linked to particular traits and health risks.

Chapter 3

The Type A Blood Diet.

It is thought that nations with a high concentration on agriculture and predominantly plant-based diets are where Type A blood first emerged. Those with Type A blood are known to have sensitive immune systems and are more prone to diseases like heart disease, diabetes, and cancer that are brought on by stress. Also, they typically have lower stomach acid levels, which makes it more difficult to digest meat.

The Recommended Diet For Type A People Is Explained As Follows:

The ideal diet for Type A people is largely vegetarian and consists of whole, organic, and freshly prepared meals. It places a strong emphasis on a selection of fruits, vegetables, grains, legumes, and nuts. In moderation, lean proteins like fish, turkey, and chicken are also acceptable.

Dietary Benefits For Type A:
There are a number of potential health advantages to the Type A diet, including:

Weight Loss: The diet's high fiber content and low saturated fat content can aid in weight loss.

Better Digestion: The Type A diet promotes the eating of whole, organic, fresh foods, which can help with digestion and relieve gastrointestinal problems.

Decreased Inflammation: Fruits and vegetables, which are high in anti-inflammatory nutrients, can help reduce inflammation in the body.

Reduced Risk Of Heart Disease: The Type A diet places an emphasis on healthy fats like those found in fish, nuts, and seeds, which can help lower the risk of heart disease. The Type A diet is low in saturated fat.

Improved energy: The Type A diet has a strong emphasis on whole, fresh, and organic foods, which can provide you with consistent energy all day.

Items To Stay Away From On A Type A Diet:
Some items should be avoided in order to maximize the advantages of the Type A diet, including:

Meat: Type A people typically have lower stomach acid levels, which makes it more difficult to digest meat.

Dairy: Some Type A people may have trouble digesting dairy products, which are thought to contribute to the creation of mucus.

Wheat: Wheat contains a protein called gluten, which some Type A people may find challenging to digest.

Processed And Refined Foods: These foods have minimal nutritional value and are heavy in sugar, salt, and harmful fats.

Certain Veggies: Several vegetables, including tomatoes, eggplants, and peppers, can irritate some Type A people.

The Type A diet is predominantly vegetarian and places an emphasis on whole, fresh, and organic foods. It is thought to have a number of health advantages, including greater energy, improved digestion, lowered risk of heart disease, reduced inflammation, and weight loss.

Type A people can maximize the advantages of the diet and enhance their general health and wellness by avoiding specific foods including meat, dairy, wheat, processed and refined foods, and some vegetables.

Chapter 4

The Type B Diet.

Red blood cells with the B antigen present on their surface are considered to be blood type B. People with type B blood have distinctive characteristics that set them different from people with other blood types. The blood type diet idea contends that type B people have more adaptable digestive systems and can tolerate a wider range of foods. They are believed to have descended from nomadic tribes that consumed both plants and animals as part of their diet.

A Detailed Explanation Of The Type B Diet Recommendation:

A mix of both plant-based and animal-based foods is encouraged by the Type B diet. Diets high in green vegetables, eggs, low-fat dairy products, lean meats like lamb and rabbit, and fish like salmon and cod are advised for Type B people. In moderation, they can also eat some cereals, nuts, seeds, and fruits.

Where possible, the Type B diet emphasizes the value of consuming organic, fresh, and locally sourced foods. In order to keep their blood sugar levels consistent, Type B people should eat a few smaller meals throughout the day rather than three large ones.

Dietary Benefits For Type B:

For people with this blood type, the Type B diet is thought to offer a host of health advantages. Improved digestion, more energy, better mental clarity, and a stronger immune system are a few of these advantages. It is also believed to lower the risk of contracting illnesses including diabetes, cancer, and heart disease.

Foods To Stay Away From On The Type B Diet:

The blood type diet idea states that Type B people should steer clear of some foods that may have a negative impact on their health. Among the foods that are advised to be avoided are:

Red Meat: Those with type B should stay away from eating red meat, especially hog, beef, and chicken. Some meats are thought to contain lectins that agglutinate and can upset the stomach.

Wheat: Those with type B diabetes are recommended to stay away from foods containing wheat, such as bread, pasta, and cereal. It is thought that wheat causes stomach problems by causing inflammation in the digestive tract.

Corn: Type B people should stay away from corn and corn-based items including popcorn, corn syrup, and cornmeal. It is thought that lectins found in corn can agglutinate Type B blood cells.

Tomatoes: Those with Type B digestion are recommended to stay away from tomatoes as they may cause problems.

Shellfish: Because they can trigger allergic reactions in some people with type B, shellfish like shrimp, crab, and lobster should be avoided.

A balanced diet known as the type B diet consists of a variety of foods from both plant and animal sources. It emphasizes the need of eating locally farmed foods that are fresh and avoiding specific meals that may be unhealthy. The blood type diet notion is unsupported by scientific research, yet people of all blood types can benefit greatly from eating a balanced, healthful diet.

Chapter 5

Type AB Diet.

The most uncommon blood type, type AB, is thought to have traits of both blood types A and B. This indicates that people with Type AB blood have certain nutritional needs that distinguish them apart from people with other blood types.

It is thought that a combination of Type A and Type B blood types is where Type AB blood got its start. Red blood cells from people with Type AB blood contain both A and B antigens, and the plasma also contains both A and B antibodies. Because of this, people with Type AB blood have unique immunological and digestive systems.

A Detailed Explanation Of The Diet For Type AB People.

The Type A and Type B diets are combined to create the Type AB diet. Its foundation is the notion that people with Type AB should follow a balanced diet consisting of a variety of foods. Lean protein, veggies, and whole grains are prioritized in the diet. Some of the meals that are advised for Type AB people include:

Lean meats like turkey, tofu, and seafood

vegetables like kale, broccoli, and spinach

Healthy grains like quinoa and brown rice

berries, plums, and kiwis, among other fruits

dairy food like kefir and yogurt

The Type AB Diet's Advantages:
The Type AB diet is thought to have a number of health advantages for those with Type AB blood types. The following are a few advantages of this diet:

Better Digestion: The Type AB diet is intended to support normal digestion and lower the risk of digestive problems including bloating and gas.

Weight Loss: The Type AB diet has a strong emphasis on veggies and lean proteins, which can help people with this blood type lose weight and keep it off.

Improved Immune System Performance: The Type AB diet is full of nutrients and antioxidants that can strengthen the immune system and lower the risk of infections and diseases.

Items To Steer Clear Of On A Type AB Diet:

Foods that are incompatible with blood type AB should be avoided by those with that blood type. On the Type AB diet, some items should be avoided, such as:

Red Meat: Those with type AB should avoid eating a lot of red meat because it can be hard to digest and raise the risk of digestive problems.

Dairy Goods: For Type AB people, some dairy items, like cheese and milk, may cause stomach problems. Processed and refined foods should be avoided by Type AB people since they may include additives and preservatives that are bad for their health.

The Type AB diet is created to offer people with Type AB blood types a nutritious and balanced diet that is suitable for their particular immune and digestive systems. People can improve their digestion, keep a healthy weight, and strengthen their immune systems by adhering to the Type AB diet.

Chapter 6

The Type O Diet.

Type O blood is the most common and oldest blood type. It is believed that those with Type O blood are descended from hunters and gatherers who mostly ate meat, fish, and vegetables. As a result, Type O people have distinct dietary requirements that are different from those of people with other blood types.

For those with Type O, a diet that is high in protein and low in carbohydrates is advised. This indicates that grains and legumes should be avoided or consumed in moderation and that the majority of their diet should consist of meat, fish, and poultry. In addition, a diet should be abundant in fruits and vegetables, particularly those that are high in phytochemicals and antioxidants.

A Type O diet has a number of advantages. For starters, it can aid people in maintaining a healthy weight and lower their risk of contracting chronic illnesses like diabetes and heart disease. Moreover, it might enhance digestion and increase energy.

Those with Type O should, however, avoid certain items. They consist of legumes like beans, lentils, and peanuts as well as grains like wheat, corn, and barley. In those with Type O blood, these foods can contribute to inflammation and digestive problems. Dairy products should also be kept to a minimum because many Type O people have trouble digesting lactose.

The Type O diet is a distinct and specialized eating plan designed to meet the nutritional requirements of people with Type O blood. Those with Type O can lower their chance of acquiring chronic diseases and enhance their general health and well-being by adhering to this diet. Hence, if you have Type O, it would be worthwhile to think about implementing some of these dietary modifications into your way of life!

Chapter 7

Personalizing Your Diet.

It might be difficult to adjust your diet, especially if you don't know where to begin. Yet, you can tailor your diet to meet your particular needs and interests with a little research and advice. Knowing your blood type and adjusting your eating habits accordingly is one method of customizing your diet.

A quick blood test is all that is necessary to determine your blood type. Once you are aware of your blood type, you can adjust your diet to meet the needs of your body. Four blood kinds exist: A, B, AB, and O. Based on the idea that various blood types are formed in various ways and have various nutritional needs, each blood type has its own set of dietary recommendations.

A diet high in fruits, vegetables, and whole grains that is plant-based may be advantageous if you have blood type A, for example. On the other hand, blood type B might respond better to a diverse diet that contains meat, dairy, and seafood. Blood type O may do well with a high-protein diet that includes meat and fish, whereas blood type AB may benefit from a combination of the A and B diets.

Adapting your diet based on your blood type might be quite advantageous. One benefit is that it can aid in weight loss and general health improvement. You may improve your digestion, metabolism, and immune system by consuming meals that are optimal for your body. Personalizing your diet can also make you feel more in touch with your body and enable you to make better food decisions.

The emotional impact that altering your diet can have on your life may be its most significant advantage. You feel in charge of your health and empowered when you consume a diet that is customized to your own needs and tastes. You may take genuine and individualized control of your well-being without having to rely on general dietary suggestions that might not work for you.

Adapting your diet based on your blood type can be a potent approach to boost your physical and mental health as well as your emotional state. You may maximize your body's performance, shed pounds, and feel more at one with your body by taking the time to find out your blood type and changing your diet accordingly. Why not attempt it then? You might feel the benefits in your body, mind, and spirit.

Chapter 8

Benefits And Drawbacks Of Blood Type Diet.

The blood type diet is a well-known eating plan that advocates for people to eat in accordance with their blood type. According to the diet, some foods are healthy for people with particular blood types while others are unhealthy. There are benefits and drawbacks to the diet, as well as critiques and restrictions.

Benefits Of The Blood Type Diet Includes:

Personalized: The blood type diet offers a dietary strategy that is specific to each individual.

Individuals can learn which foods, based on their blood type, are the most beneficial for their bodies according to the diet plan. For some people, this customized approach to diet and nutrition may be more successful than a one-size-fits-all strategy.

Weight Loss: Several people claim to have lost weight after implementing the blood-type diet. The diet's emphasis on full, nutrient-dense foods and restriction of processed and refined meals is probably to blame for this.

Better Digestion: For some people, the blood type diet may result in improved digestion. The diet places an emphasis on simple-to-digest foods and steers clear of those that could upset the stomach.

Improved Energy: Some people say that eating according to their blood type gives them more energy. This might be a result of the diet's focus on full, nutrient-dense meals, which give the body steady energy throughout the day.

Limitations Of The Blood Type Diet And Criticisms Of It.

Scientific Evidence Lacking: There isn't any evidence at this time to back up the blood type diet. There is no proof that eating in accordance with one's blood type is advantageous, despite certain research linking blood type to a connection with specific health issues.

Restrictive: For people with certain blood types, the blood type diet can be highly restrictive. This can make it challenging to maintain the diet over time and may result in vitamin shortages.

Unreliable Advice: The blood type diet offers erroneous advice for several meals. For instance, it is suggested that some blood types avoid dairy while others consume it in moderation. Those who are on a diet may find this to be puzzling.

The Danger Of Misdiagnosis: According to the blood type diet, each person has one of four blood types. There are numerous distinct blood types as well as variants within each blood type group, though. As a result, people could receive a false diagnosis and dietary guidance that is inappropriate for them.

Although the blood type diet may have certain benefits, its claims are not yet backed by any scientific data. The diet may not be suitable for everyone and can be rather restrictive. Before making any dietary changes, it is crucial to see your doctor if you are thinking about trying the blood type diet.